I0791100

Understanding And Treating ADHD

Contents

ADD: How Is It Different From ADHD?

Attention Deficit Disorder or ADD is a very complicated, and time and again misinterpreted, disorder. Its beginning is physiological, but it can have a multitude of consequences that come alongside with it. That apart, what is the differentiation between ADHD and ADD? ADHD is the abbreviated form of Attention Deficit Hyperactive Disorder, its major indications being noticeable hyperactivity and impulsivity. These are the indications that are noticeable to the purposeful onlooker. ADD stands for Attention Deficit Disorder with the major indications being lack of concentration. Now a lot of other things can come alongside with both of these subtypes of ADHD, but those are the distinctive characteristics of both.

For several years, the usual picture of Attention Deficit Disorder has been the little boy that is bouncing off the walls and making his teachers and parents go mad. ADHD is beyond a doubt the more identifiable of the two subtypes since it is so much more noticeable than ADD. Since hyperactivity causes a lot more disruption and problems for classrooms, it gets the most notice and will be picked up on a lot quicker. Unluckily, even if ADD is less visible, the consequences of the disorder can just as negative.

With negligent attention deficit disorder, or ADD, the person enduring it will give the impression of being spacey and disordered. More often, victims with this type will be gazing out of the window during classes and will seem as if they are never somewhat there. It is much more tricky to make a diagnosis and a lot of people with this form of ADD go years without even knowing they have it. But the consequences of the drifting mind can be just as disparaging.

For a long time, it was considered that only boys suffered from ADHD. However, this figment has been busted of late. It is now acknowledged that both girls and boys can suffer from attention deficit disorder, and many do not get out of it in middle age. One disparity that has been noticed is that girls are inclined to have the inattentive version of ADD, and many times it is wrongly diagnosed as depression. Since inattentive ADD does not create noticeable troubles and disruptions to the nearby surroundings, a lot of them endure in silence for years before they discover the real reason of their plight.

With both ADHD and ADD, making a diagnosis early on is very essential. Even though troubles with schools are the most apparent indications, some victims do not have major problems with

Understanding And Treating ADHD

getting school work completed. Keep track of your children, not just academically, but generally and psychologically as well. Do they have problem with other children? Does it appear as if they have difficulty putting in order or are extremely disordered? Do they have difficulty sitting motionless for a period of time? Are they extremely silent or extremely chatty? Now any of these indications do not in particular denote ADD or ADHD, but they do point to asking for outside help from a therapist or a counselor.

Your child's psychological well being is just as vital as their physical well being and how they do in school. Confirm it out if you sense like something is off. If left for years not diagnosed, ADD can create a lot of other resulting troubles that can take a long time to get rid off and can be arrested.

ADD: The Types Of Its Manifestation In Kids

Attention Deficit Disorder can take several forms in children. It is not difficult to track the child with ADD who is very chaotic. Boys generally come into this category. But then there are some types of ADD which go undiagnosed because their effects in children are less outwardly evident. This happens mainly in case of girls.

There are many girls who are called "tomboys". They frequently exhibit some of the important features off ADD, like being more involved in physical activities, but not as reckless as the boys themselves. As a result teachers and parents jump to the conclusion that the child has no interest in academics and is basically not organized, but the possibility of ADD is seldom considered.

Besides the "tomboy" types, the "chatty" girls could also be suffering from ADD, but remaining undiagnosed. This is a fusion of over-activity and inattentiveness, and is usually touted as socially extrovert. These girls are extremely talkative than being physically active and cannot stop talking even if they are strictly warned. They also cannot tell stories comprehensively and will stray from their thoughts because of ADD.

Those whom we call as "daydreamers" could also be suffering from ADD. They do not draw any attention to themselves and are very quite in nature. However, their too much being into themselves and not giving any attention to the class is another form of ADD, contrary to the "chatty" girls. They may show anxiety and depression when given school projects, but cannot finish the projects because of their lack of staying power. This generally goes undiagnosed because the child is thought to be lazy and, parents and teachers fail to identify the disorder in time.

What is fascinating is that many girls with ADD have quite a high rate of IQ and could be called "gifted". When a child has a high IQ there are no problems in school work, but their lack loopholes get reflected as they mature into adults. Keep in mind that ADD is not a learning disorder, and patients do not inevitably are poor performers in school. Till high school they can be quite well off, but with mounting pressure and assignments symptoms may become more and more evident.

Understanding And Treating ADHD

When undiagnosed, Attention Deficit Disorder may cause a lot of harm to an individual. Children will be called unorganized, lacking intelligence and lazy, when in truth, they might be silent sufferers of ADD. They will have very low esteem of themselves, and believe themselves to be quitters or stupid because of their problems. It is crucial that the problem is identifies and treated before it becomes too late and any long-term damage is done.

Attention Deficit Disorder: Getting Your Facts Right

With all that is written about ADHD, most of us tend to think of a bad little lad running about ruining whatever comes his way. So we often believe that we can spot the child with ADD while we are out. Well the naughty little boy is there fine, but did we ever spare a thought about the little girl who sits quiet and withdrawn with her mother, one who is overtly polite, terribly afraid to speak out and draws a blank when spoken to? In all probabilities, everyone would fail to guess that she might be suffering from ADD or the Attention Deficit Disorder.

Difficult as they are, ADD and ADHD have some obvious symptoms too. The affected person suffers from distraction, easy forgetfulness and low self-esteem, faces problem in following fast conversations and gets highly disordered with tasks. ADD and ADHD both can retard mental growth in this that the affected child has to struggle with school work and assignment deadlines, failing to finish things on time. These disorders also rob the child off his/her ability to manage the belongings and to keep track of time.

ADD Symptoms:

- Lacks vigor, suffers from sloth
- Values others more, respecting their individual limits
- Often unassertive or under-assertive
- Too much obedience
- Excessive humbleness and modesty
- Overtly polite and shy
- Avoiding crowd, preferring to stay alone and socially withdrawn
- Not able to open up easily and befriend, although they make a few bonds

Since it is assumed that girls are generally shy, people often overlook the ADD symptoms in them and they are left untreated. Their outward calm, quiet and politeness are usually to cover up the inner disturbance. ADD affected girls are emotional and highly sensitive to criticism; but the feelings invoked thus, after being criticized, remain untold. They just carry on with life, struggling silently. Interestingly enough, their ADHD counterparts move forward with absolutely no sign of stress or fatigue and seem totally unaffected by all deterrents in the walk of life. Girls suffering from ADD cannot withstand stress and usually draw back more into a shell with a belief that they are good-for-nothing and can never do anything right.

Helping a person with ADD

All ADD affected girls are predominantly emotional, irrespective of their nature—be it shy, social, introvert, hyperactive or super-impulsive. This over-sensitivity evidently invites regular upsets which, in turn, give rise to more and more stress. Hence, they should be taught to manage stress through various techniques from an early age. They must also be ascribed a certain revival time to regroup or collect themselves after every damage or emotional upset.

Although it is true that parents always wish the best for their children, they sometimes, unknowingly, impede mental growth in their kids by hurling too much criticism at them or by driving them mad with a series of never-ending do's and don'ts like "You must not be so silly. You got to finish school with high grades", "You need to improve your looks. Try and be as smart as your brother", "You should be a little more assertive. This won't help", "why do you let yourself be taken for granted? Wake up", "Make more friends", "Do not let go off things so easily" so on and so forth. While all these are fine at times, too much of criticism breeds low self-esteem in her—be she shy, outspoken, drawn-back or unruly!

At school, throughout the day, the confidence and self-regard of these girls are constantly shattered and their only respite is at home, where they can rebuild their crushed dignity and revitalize themselves to fight another day. Continuous criticism roots in them the belief that they are worthless. These girls suffering from ADD become extremely impulsive, disorganized and lack focus in everything only to secure poor grades in class. Full of distractions, these girls lack the vigor and energy to develop their personality and skill sets that their peers have. Instead of pointing at their limitations, it is better to compliment them or appreciate when they pick up a skill or show signs of a good ability. Their psyche just needs a positive boost. And it's not hard to make them feel good—an ADD-affected girl can easily get lucky and find interest in some activity. That then becomes the first positive move, the most desired turning point in their lives!

Attention Deficit Disorder: Is It Really That?

Attention Deficit Disorder or ADD is most frequently identified in boys of primary school age. Indications consist of lack of concentration, being restless, reckless mannerisms, or lack of focus. But what brings about these indications, in fact? And should every one of the occurrences of ADD be treated?

In a few occurrences, the indications of ADD may in fact be indicative of a more severe psychological predicament, such as depression, bipolar disorder, brain defects and even nervousness. On the other hand, at times the occurrence of the particular inattentive behavior may simply be due to allergic reactions, sensitivities to the environment, nutritional deficits or also too much caffeine.

Many times, young boys are wrongly diagnosed with Attention Deficit Disorder merely for conducting themselves the way anybody would be expecting. Young boys will by and large make reckless resolutions, have a lot of superfluous energy, cannot sit still, and have short concentration period in school. Combined with the fact that the majority of school age children use up more than forty hours a week watching TV and playing computer games, it is not a surprise that a lot of children have energy to use up.

ADD mannerism is frequently indicative of creativeness, giftedness, high aptitude, and a child being a visual theorist.

In short, an analysis of Attention Deficit Disorder ought to be thought of as a start, and not an end. Too frequently, when a doctor sees that a child is agitated and has a short concentration period, she writes a medication for Dexedrine or Ritalin and that is that. But these drugs have possibly unsafe side effects, and are not essentially going to cure the predicament at all.

A further comprehensive examination of the occurrence generally falls upon the child's parents. The facts stated here is aimed to steer the parents in the right track, giving propositions of where to begin looking for the reason of the child's Attention Deficit Disorder related manners.

Attention Deficit Hyperactivity Disorder: What Is It?

Attention Deficit Hyperactivity Disorder or ADHD is a mental disorder, which approximately three to seven percent children are having. Due to this disorder children manifest the characteristic of constant behavior, loads of activity as well as often being considered disobedient. That does not mean that the individual is being bad but the thing is, they don't have control over their mental range. They go through lack of concentration because at a time they are likely to be thinking about many elements instead of one particular element.

This disorder is also found in many adults besides children. In adults, it is called Adult Attention Deficit Disorder or AADD. Among all children diagnosed with ADHD about 30 to 70 percent will carry on with their disorder through adulthood. Adults learn to live with it and work around it and need less help. They can handle the disorder of their own and so it's harder to detect also. Yet, in many cases both children and adult may need medications for better results.

In children this disorder shows signs like inattentiveness, impulsive behavior and a constant restlessness. In adults, it is harder to diagnose but children with this disorder cannot sit still for long. They cannot concentrate on one particular thing for a long period of time. In adults, it becomes difficult sometimes to structure their lives and to plan daily activities. They don't feel the importance to stay attentive or to stop being restless because these are not at all important problems for them.

ADHD is a disorder for which assistance of medical personnel is necessary. It can be treated but cannot be cured fully. For this disorder medication is also necessary.

6 Tips For Slowing Down The ADD Brain

If you are an adult suffering with ADD, then you might recognize that although it is easy to say, slowing down can be a very difficult if not impossible thing to do at first glance.

No matter who you are there are numerous things that have to be done and all too often little time available to get them done. So then your mind starts to work at high speed in an attempt to achieve as much as it can and more. The result can be stress at not being able to meet your requirements, leading to you getting upset about the fact that it looks impossible. Because of this you use up lots of time worrying, and unfortunately little time enjoying yourself.

Whilst slowing down can be a complex thing to achieve it can be done. Here are six established methods to assist you to slow your brain ADD or otherwise:

1. Put down your work

Set business hours and no matter what is left at the end of the day, walk away. Stand by your rules. Even though it is going to seem necessary to work overtime, avoid it at all cost. You will work better and more efficiently during the shorter hours of the day knowing that you must leave at a set time. And take weekends (or at least a couple of days a week off).

2. Commit to a regular obligation

Commit to a reason to get out of your house or out of your office each week. You may want to attend a class, possibly something that you have always wanted to do. Make sure that you 'pay' in advance for the class so that you have a reason to attend.

3. Arrange for a break with others

Few things are as enjoyable as having a night out with friends. This may be with colleagues, with friends, with family, or with members of another group.

4. Keep a diary

Writing in a diary requires that you stop, think about what you want to say, and then act on what you think. It helps you to deal with nervous tension and achieve clearness. make a resolution to write every day - even if only for a few minutes!

5. Switch your computer off two hours before bed

Because computers are an access point to interesting things, for ADDers you can find yourself sitting at a computer until the early hours of the morning completely oblivious to what is happening around you. To make sure that this doesn't happen to you switch the computer off at least 2 hours before you plan to go to sleep so as to suitably relax and slow down at night.

6. Meditate

There are diverse methods of meditation, so find one that suits you, but you may want to consider mindfulness meditation. This is the action of keeping your mind in the present - whether you are walking, working or washing dishes. Make an effort to keep your mind in the here and now not the past or future.

It is fine to start doing this little by little, with short sessions spent in mindful meditation daily (possibly only 5 minutes at a time), after that building your performance as you become more at ease.

Attention Deficit Disorder: What Is It Anyway?

As parents, I am sure that many of you will have spent sleepless nights concerned that the strange behavior our child exhibited today may be the first signs of Attention Deficit Disorder. Our concerns are justified in many ways as most of us believe we know the fundamental signs of the disease are, and we obviously panic at the thought we might have to deal with it.

The fear of the disease, its effects and the way it will impact on the family is only one part of it. There is often an underlying guilt that in some way our actions may be responsible for this having happened. Most of us will in some way or another blame ourselves, believing that we have not been strict enough or applied enough discipline, or conversely that we have been too strict. While these apprehensions may be quite normal the ideas aren't always rational or well-founded.

There are usually assed to be three broad stages in any normal childhood development;

The first is observable in babies / infants. During this stage infants become focused on and preoccupied with certain objects to the exclusion of what else is around them. If a kid's development stalls around this point it may later show as signs of autism.

In the second recognizable stage, which is observed in older children, the child becomes interested in a range of things at the same time and they then become incapable of concentrating or focusing on any one thing or action for any length of time. This is the key to ADD, as If the child stalls in their development at this stage they may later in their childhood go on to suffer Attention Deficit Disorder (ADD).

The third stage assists a child to mature to a point from which they can comfortably focus and voluntarily apply their attention in one certain direction for longer periods of time. They can then alter their focus or actions as and when they have a need to. This stage is therefore a crucial transitional stage which moulds a child for success in the classroom and in the real world.

But ADD does not only make a child or young adult incapable of focusing. It also reduces their ability to take decisions. They can then become indecisive even in normal everyday life. An

Understanding And Treating ADHD

example may be that they become disoriented when crossing a road and turn back into on-coming traffic, or lose the reason why they were crossing in the first place.

At the opposite end of the scale, ADD sufferers can also become totally focused on a specific object or task. They can become consumed by it and are as a result are absolutely cut-off and oblivious to everything else. an example of this manifesting is that they may watch the same movie again and again without realizing, or read a certain part of a book repeatedly with no reaction or loss of concentration. Later in life this behavior might turn into over-eating or substance-abuse or other compulsive behavior.

Another increasingly reported variation of ADD is Attention Deficit Hyperactivity Disorder known as ADHD. This leads to sufferers always needing to stay busy, moving from place to place or being unable to slow down. It is increasingly being diagnosed in young teenagers. This can drive parents mad and keep them up nights in an attempt to calm their child and entice them to sleep. These children and young adults will find it difficult to switch off but they can experience many of the events above. While experience of this type of patient has led Psychologists to conclude that ADD is not a problem that a child will grow out of naturally they have also quite strongly rejected any link with the parent causing this disorder. There is no direct causal relationship between what a parent does an how likely a child is to develop ADD or ADHD. So if your child is suffering from ADD stop blaming yourself, instead recognize the problem for what it is and contact a specialist as soon as possible.

ADD: How Does It Affect Your Child's Schooling And Education?

There is no doubt that it is a difficult task to teach any child, but more so one suffering from Attention Deficit Disorder. A significant number of schools have identified ADD as a legitimate problem and have ADDressed the issue with changes in teaching methods. Substantial developments and improvements have been made in methodology to recognize the disorder, but there are still some which lag behind in arrangements and cannot answer an individual's needs.

The way in which ADD can influence a classroom is often seen even before a diagnosis has been made. It might be observed in a child reacting to his classmates, as physical reactions such as snatching books, or in a child sitting in a corner, her mind elsewhere.

It is often a teacher who recognizes that a student is having problems attending to lessons or are over-active. But identifying the problem is just the first step, the most difficult thing is changing the behavior.

The treatment of ADD can only start once everyone acknowledges it. Then a diagnosis has to be made before a course of treatment is agreed. It is important early in the day to decide if medicine as a method is required, since this will determine the course of any treatment. There are some schools, which insist that a child suffering with ADD be given medicines to mitigate the effects. Some schools, however take a more patient stance and are wiling to comply with the parent's wishes.

In an ideal world, your child should be in a school which understands the effectiveness that working together as part of a team causes, by the school administration taking involvement in your child's circumstances and respecting decisions as a parent. This will assist your child in achieving the best that they can.

Regrettably some schools do not have such an open-minded vision. Communities which are smaller, and places which are poorer relative to other districts may have a habit of being too conservative. These schools can sometimes lag in catering to children who have a special need or suffer from a specific situation.

Understanding And Treating ADHD

ADD does make some children harder to teach. They are often more chaotic and more difficult to control. For these reasons a few schools refuse to take on and accommodate such potentially unruly children. Regardless of this you must make sure that no child is provided with a sub-standard, second-rate treatment under any circumstances.

As well as the above, some schools may run remedial classes, or classes only for students with learning issues. Rather than these classes always assisting such children, they can be disadvantaged by this. Children with ADD are not necessarily less intelligent at all, but classes such as these are often of mixed abilities.

Remember though that you are the parent. You have the responsibility to achieve the best for your child. You should always be there for him or her. If any decision taken by the school of the class teacher goes against what you perceive to be the well-being or the best education for your child, you should immediately discuss it with them. You may be able to come to a better plan that will ensure the best for your child.

ADD And The Gift Of Resilience

Attention Deficit Disorder creates diverse tests for different people. It is not uncommon for people to struggle when trying to work, whether for a lack of attention, too many interesting distractions or something else. When you have ADD it is so much harder to overcome these factors, but there is one way that is guaranteed to help - develop the ability to be tough and determined.

Resilience is defined as 'the ability to recover from or adjust easily to changes or misfortune.' When relating this to adults with ADD, we need to adapt the description slightly to be 'an ability to adjust to adversity without difficulty, to make progress when faced with change, to overcome hold ups, challenges or disappointments.'

In order to develop as adults with ADD, we must acknowledge the inevitable - that we will be faced with problems, that we will experience disappointments and frustrations. But that said we cannot allow these to stop us.

We can take a real look at an example of how resilience applies by evaluating two adults with ADD, Julie and Sally.

Julie is a very smart woman, but does not think of herself in that way. She works in a high pressure office where people are very active, verging on hyperactive. She works as general assistant to a number of VIPs. One of those she works for often blames his mistakes on her, while another boss repeatedly calls Julie unintelligent.

She spends her evenings thinking of her failings, exhausted and distressed. As a result she feels overwhelmed. While she had once been a very positive, cheerful woman, she has now let the comments of a few people bring her down. While she wishes to look for a new job she doubts that anyone will employ her.

Sally is also a smart woman suffering from ADD. She had a difficult time at school, did not achieve very good grades, and was repeatedly told she was lazy, but she persisted. She graduated from high school and, even though her parents dissuaded her from going to college, she went anyway. She started in community college. When she found that she could choose her own courses of study, she did pretty well.

Sally was determined to teach high school as she wanted to provide a positive influence on the people around her - especially other kids. Her college counselor had told her that she was foolish to even think of it. The counselor had told her that '...a person like you will not be able to teach high school. You will not be able to control the children.'

Sally was disappointed for a couple of days but deep down in her heart, she knew different. She chose not to pay attention to her counselor and instead she formally requested a different career's counselor complaining that she should have a person who would provide encouragement. And she was placed with one who then reassessed her needs and was more supportive.

Sally is now teaching high school history and has been for 7 years. She has been nominated for numerous awards and has been awarded 'Best High School Teacher' twice.

Julie has lost her determination because of what has happened to her. She has allowed the negative impressions of others to change her opinions about her own worth and her ability and she no more belief in herself.

Sally, on the other hand, has retained her remarkable determination. And through it all she has believed in herself. She does not let the views or misconceptions of others' bring her down. She allows herself to reflect and to be sADDened but not for long.

Resilience in adults with ADD is all about moving ahead. If we would like to be flourishing grown ups with ADD, we cannot allow setbacks to hold us back.

ADHD: How To Plan Your Child's Treatment Successfully

Assuming that you have already taken your child or teenager to a behavioral specialist and had their actions evaluated by an expert you should now be aware of the problems you face. But at least if you now know that you are faced with ADHD you should be on the way to developing a decent treatment plan.

Quite rightly, your child's psychologist, therapist or physician should now want to start out on a course of treatment . But what do you need to know before you agree to sign off on and agree to any specific course of action? How do you know that what they come up with is beneficial and the best option?

Here are a few propositions for you to think on. What is listed below are only our ideas, but these have been formulated after having worked with over 1,000 children, young adults and teenagers with diagnosed ADHD (attention deficit hyperactivity disorder).

1. Make use of all of your opinions. Have a detailed discussion with a physician, ideally your family doctor but do not be stonewalled by them. Any recommended course of action should be well reasoned and will differ child by child.

2. Through summer holiday we like to use "alternative" treatments such as homeopathy, manipulating diet using our suggested eating plans, and increasing the consumption of essential fatty acid supplements.

3. EEG Biofeedback training has also been found to offer excellent results and should be seen as an "alternative" healing method for ADD. The benefit of this is that if these treatments are effective (and in our experience they are almost 70% of the time) then we can keep the patient away from chemical treatments.

If the initial analysis and diagnosis is made later in a school year then we tend to suggest a medical treatment right away for almost all patients. When summer approaches we would attempt to reduce dosage of medicines and try the methods above. The reason we would use a chemical treatment is to try to 'salvage' the school year. ADHD may result in a worsening

Understanding And Treating ADHD

school performance. Since medicines tend to work quickly, the student may be able to get through and pass classes they might otherwise fail.

In Addition to this, by trying out the medicines ahead of the summer we have something to benchmark against. We can compare the results of chemical medical solutions to other less invasive treatments to be tried and tested during the summer holidays.

It is worth bearing in mind that physicians and not always open-minded when looking at alternative medicines. Doctors tend to utilize what they know - chemical medical solutions - without being willing in some cases to examine alternatives. Make sure that when you go to them you are fully versed in what you want and do not let yourself be swayed easily by their recalcitrance.

I did this myself for many years, and this is where you have got to come to a decision yourself on how best to help your child or teenager with Attention Deficit Disorder.

An Introduction To Attention Deficit Hyperactivity Disorder

ADHD has many forms and numerous slightly differing manifestations. There are already more than five recorded and documented forms of ADHD.

And although sometimes questioned, it is widely acknowledged that this is a medical condition which is carried through the genes, and therefore often manifests itself as certain disorders of the nervous system (of which there are many).

The DSM-IV Manual of Diagnosis reports that any type, form or kind of Attention Deficit Hyperactivity Disorder should be grouped under the category of ADHD. This main central list is subsequently broken into ADHD types;

- ADHD Combined Type
- Impulsive-Hyperactive Type or
- ADHD Inattentive Type

Some time ago, the phrases attention deficit disorder "with" or "without" hyperactivity were also coined and widely used. There can be many combinations so that different sufferers will show different symptoms.

Generally Attention Deficit Hyperactivity affects numerous sections of the brain, often more than four unique parts of the brain. Because of this, it results in many unique "profiles" and "styles" of young people, so having a 'standard set of behavior and monitoring against that for any child and possibly even adults with ADHD or ADD doesn't always work.

There are four main spheres:

1) Inability to attend
2) Difficulties with Impulse Control
3) Problems associated with motor restlessness and/or hyperactivity
4) An increased propensity to become bored - A condition yet to be "officially" declared in manuals of diagnosis

Understanding And Treating ADHD

Here are a few more important elements of this condition:

a. When you know what to look for, this disorder and its effects are observable and can be monitored in most circumstances, but this should be done both at school and at home. If a child shows symptoms only in one place then possibly there is a reason for this which should be investigated.

b. often, the disorder becomes more noticeable before the child reaches seven years of age. Since ADHD is caused at least in part by neurological problems, it may be from a head injury or may have been carried in the genetics itself.

If ADHD is going to occur normally it will be apparent by the age of seven.

What Is It Like To Live With Attention Deficit Disorder?

Living with ADD may not be easy for any child, teenager or adult who has been diagnosed with ADD. A person recently diagnosed with ADD and predicting the rest of their life may not be easy for them. They may be unsure how their ailment will be affected by age. But as time passes and you mature with your knowledge, you start to understand ways to handle the symptoms of and effectively deal with ADD.

Children with ADD can be forgetful, ignorant of the effects of their actions on others and reckless, or they may easily get distracted. They might show too many of their feelings or activity to others. And, the symptoms will remain quite consistent even when they pass through other ages. However their ability to manage these symptoms will improve over time, as they get older.

The way ADD can impact on your life will largely be determined by what medication you select to treat the disorder. You might wish to consult a doctor to give yourself a better understanding of the future effects that taking stimulants might have, and also other implications of taking medicines.

There are many characteristics and traits which are typical of ADD. People suffering from it should be prepared for these. These might be difficulties in their being overly attentive to details, or problem with remaining calm and for any length of time. They might be fidgety or have problems being able to push on through and complete any given task.

Nevertheless it is possible to do a range of things to mitigate the behavior so often related to ADD. It is possible to become more organized and more controlled in keeping things under control. You can choose any book or a calendar in order to assist you, but the process is what is important.

Routines, schedules and planning should be used widely as these will teach you control. As a sufferer of ADD you will be naturally inclined to forget, lose control and be careless. By using a simple device such as a calendar you will behave in a more controlled manner, in a way unlike your true nature. Thus you will make less mistakes.

Understanding And Treating ADHD

You might also wish to become a part of a group as this will provide Additional support. You may feel the need for someone to confide in, who can understand you situation well. A person with ADD could be a perfect companion since they may be able to connect with you better than any friend or a family member, since they can support you only to a limit.

Attention Deficit Hyperactivity Disorder The Alternative Treatments Available

The movement away from using stimulants and medication that includes stimulants for the treatment of ADHD has resulted in a growing market for alternative treatments. Attention Deficit Hyperactivity Disorder has grown massively as a recognized illness in the past twenty years. What is surprising is that there is still a limited amount of treatments available which could be classed as 'alternative'. What follows are four powerful non-medical treatments.

1. Brainwave Bio-feedback Training
2. Behavior Modification Therapy
3. Eating / Diet Interventions
4. Nutraceutical Medicines known as Extress and Attend

These therapies can be very helpful and give significant advantages in some situations. They are excellent when combined with the expertise of a counselor who has experience working with ADD and ADHD. Unfortunately many counselors will have little knowledge of working with people with these disorders.

"Attend" and "Extress" have both been found to be superb substitutes for stimulant treatment medicines. Both of these are complicated procedures, engineered so as to achieve optimum efficiency in brain activity in individuals experiencing problems with concentration, with overcoming rage, with impulse control, with listening and paying attention, or with hyperactivity.

EEG Biofeedback training which is also known to many as Neuro feedback, has been around for at least twenty years. In that sense it may be seen by some as old technology, but it has not stood still in that time. With the development of super fast computers the technology has grown into a recognized alternative treatment for healing of ADD. And over the time it has taken to enhance the methods, a huge amount of study has taken place into EEG Biofeedback. There are many websites and a wealth of information available on this including EEG Spectrum, and other treatment alternatives are also documented well.

Eating plans and diet improvements can also have significant constructive effects on people with ADD or with Attention Deficit Hyperactivity Disorder. Even though we are reluctant to

Understanding And Treating ADHD

accept that this involvement can be applied as effectively overall as either Attend and Extress, or a session of EEG Biofeedback methods, we certainly do consider that each person with ADHD should try diet involvement.

A lot of people with ADD and ADHD will be assisted by nutritional supplements. Among the most effective supplements are often Essential Fatty Acids also often known as Omega Oils. It is also important to use supplementary minerals such as Zinc. The "Attend" nutraceutical will provide the necessary fatty acids. You also get them in Borage Oil or Flax Seed Oil. They can in Addition be found in fish, and you can just give your child more of tuna fish to eat.

How Is Attention Deficit Disorder (ADD) Diagnosed?

When assessing whether an individual suffers with Attention Deficit Disorder or not it is a lot harder than it may appear to laymen such as ourselves. The symptoms of ADD are the same as those of other ailments such as hyperthyroidism etc. Many of the symptoms are shared by all people at some point or another, so it is often the scale of these which diagnoses a person as having ADD. So the first important step in diagnosing the disease is to consult a medically trained health provider regarding it.

Because what is interpreted as Attention Deficit Disorder is still vague, diagnosing the ailment is very difficult since there is nothing which is solely a part of, or totally outside of the scope of ADD. Although various organizations such as The American Pediatrics Clinical Practice have tried to put in place guidelines in order to assist people in recognizing the disease most people including medical professionals are still often unsure about such methods.

While doctors in the past have tried to use MRI (or magnetic resonance imagery) to analyze a patient's brain to detect early signs of ADD, most medical professionals not longer recommend this. Thus diagnosis is often now based primarily on reports of people close to the patient, those who see, talk to, work or live with them and have come to understand the patient's habits well.

Guideline published by the AAP (The American Academy of Pediatrics) requires that medical personnel look into a child's behavior getting information from more than one location before they reach a conclusion as to whether or not a child is suffering from ADD. The doctor is therefore expected to need to consult various sources regarding his patient's behavior from his school, home, the playground etc. to make sure that any diagnosis is not based on a child's behavior at one place. This is so that we can know for definite that the problem is intrinsic to the child's normal personality and not just a reaction to what may have happened in one place.

The guideline also demands that a physician use "explicit criteria for diagnosis" using a DS-IV-TR standard.

Therefore when approaching a medical professional for treatment, make sure that they closely follow the directions as set by the Academy before they try to diagnose the problem.

Understanding And Treating ADHD

Remember that a problem like ADD may not be so difficult to set about curing as it is to diagnose. But proper diagnosis is likely to be a first step in a satisfactory cure.

This is a disease which is very widespread in one form or another, and is seen in differing degrees among many youngsters. While we choose to ignore the problem and deny its presence, It is am ailment which will stay with your child until they are much older, possibly for life. Therefore recognize the disease early and take your child to a medical professional for a competent diagnosis and a cure.

What Does A Diagnosis Of Attention Deficit Disorder Really Mean?

About thirty years back, a child was a born voyager, rambunctious, or was said to have been gifted with great creativity or brainpower, if he seemed to be lacking concentration, and was impatient, and impulsive. These children, due to their lack in concentration at school, were often jumped ahead, since it was thought that the work was not testing enough to match their capabilities.

However, now when a child shows these symptoms, they are generally diagnosed with ADD, i.e., Attention Deficit Disorder, and are treated as soon as possible.

ADD is quite a new discovery, and is most commonly found among elementary school boys. A typical young boy would be seen to act on impulse, have too much energy, be restless, and having a problem with concentrating in the class. Moreover, these kids usually tend to spend 40-plus hours a week, in front of the television, or playing video games. It cannot be denied that many children do have a lot of vigor.

This distracted behavior can be caused in children due to various reasons. In some cases, these factors might be quite serious, and might not have anything to do with the psychology of the child, or the child's fitness conditions. For example, the behavior usually observed in children, suffering from ADD, may be caused due to problems of child abuse or due to neglect. Usually, once a child is diagnosed with ADD, a drug like Ritalin is prescribed, and the child abuse is continued without interference.

The ADD symptoms may signify some severe psychological problems, such as the bipolar disorder, deep anxiety or depression or even defects in brain. However, in some cases, the causal factors maybe quite simple, like an allergy, sensitiveness to the environment, deficiency of nutrition, or excessive caffeine intake.

Therefore, the child's parents and teachers, along with their doctors must treat ADD as a serious issue, which should be treated with not only medication but also proper investigation.

ADHD Treatment: Starting The Process

Most parents wonder about ADHD treatments. Is this something that your child needs? How can you find out and ultimately what will the treatment involve? If you are one of these individuals, looking for a means to getting your answers will be the most important aspect. In other words, treatment can only come if you seek it out yourself. The first thing you need to do is to learn if your child even has ADHD.

Diagnosis

The first step in treatment for ADHD is to find out if the child has it. As a parent, you will want to invest some time in doing research, as there is plenty of it offered to you on the web. But, you should also include your doctor in your concerns about your child's behavior. Children that often are though to have ADHD are usually misunderstood. If you find that your child is getting in trouble more than your other children, more than other children in their class or more than you think is normal, then talking to your doctor about ADHD is essential.

To get the process started, talk to your doctor about your concerns and then work to get the answers. Most of the time, children will need to be screened by their doctor physically. Then, they will talk to their social workers, psychiatrists and other professionals that are skilled in accessing ADHD cases. The testing may be just a series of questions to you and to your child individually. Encourage them to really talk about how they feel not to try to answer as they think you want to hear. In Addition to these talks, your child may be asked to listen and respond to other tests.

Since each child is quite different, the process of assessing their condition is likely to be different for each child and each doctor. In some cases, it will be necessary to determine if the child has ADHD or if they perhaps have a learning disability. Often these can be interchangeable but getting the right diagnosis means getting the right treatment so it should take a bit of an extra step if necessary.

 Once this process has been completed, you will work with your doctor to determine the right ADHD treatment for your child. It may be simple or it may be complex. Whatever it is, it is likely to be well worth the process. The fact is that your child can find relief if you get the process started.

Herbal ADHD Treatments

For those that are suffering from ADHD, there are many treatment options out there. Some people do not like to use chemical medications to treat conditions such as this. These individuals will attempt to seek out the help that they need in treating ADHD with alternative remedies. There are some wonderful herbal remedies that can help to promote health and well being to those that are looking for something other than medications. Although you should never just stop taking any type of medication prescribed to you by a doctor, you may find some relief in these herbal remedies as well.

One way to know if an herbal product has shown to be any type of help on the condition that you are faced with is to look at research studies. In some studies that have been done around the world in the last several years, there are some Chinese herbal remedies that have shown to provide children with improved well being and even treat ADD and ADHD effectively. One herbal remedy that does this includes herbal components including Chinese throwax root, skullcap root, ginseng root, red jujube fruit and other ingredients. The combination of the ingredients was said to provide a calming effect on the child.

Another formula that is used for ADHD treatment offers an anti-depressive formula and treatment. Here, you will find ingredients such as St. John's Wort, Kava Kava, Chamomile, Lavender essential oils, Skullcap, Signseng, and orange essential oil. This combination is said to provide for a treatment for ADHD as well.

Ginkgo is one herb that you may find in some of these herbal remedies. This type of herb is said to improve the blood flow to the brain. By increasing the vascular circulation there, it is said to provide improved memory as well as improving concentration. Hawthorne is another treatment options. Here, the goal is to strengthen the heart and the circulatory system. It is used in many ancient Chinese medications to calm the mind. In Addition, herbs like skullcap, lemon balm and oats are used to help provide a nerve tonic that will help to nourish as well as offer normality to the nervous system, improving the individual's overall calmness and clarity.

Herbal remedies have been used for many years to treat conditions such as ADHD. Trying to incorporate some of these remedies can often be helpful. As they are natural, they are unlikely to cause side effects to the individual as well as long as they are taken as they are directed.

ADHD Treatments: An Overview

Finding the right ADHD treatment means finding the right combination of treatment options for you. Each child or adult that has ADHD will find himself a bit unique in his situation. Just like any other condition, it is essential to gear the treatment of that condition to the specifics of it. Yet, there is an overall significant similarity between the treatments offered. That is that each diagnosis and treatment will come with medication help, behavior help as well as educational interventions.

Medications

The first thing that comes to individual's minds when they here medication is illness. The fact is that children and adults that suffer from ADHD will experience conditions that are not like others. They often see things or learn things in a unique way. Often times this learning curve is something that needs to be well understood before medications can be administered. There are many medications that are available to aid in helping the individual deal with the conditions that his or her ADHD is causing. Some are very mind, some are very strong. Some offer very few side effects, others many. Your doctor will work with you to determine the right medication for your needs.

Behavior Therapy

Teaching the child how to cope with various situations when it comes to their ADHD can be greatly appreciated. Children that understand how to react when they are frustrated, angry or misunderstood can learn to better control their behavior and then find more success in their treatment. Yet, behavior therapy is often not enough on its own. Adding medication to the process can offer more rewards.

Educational Intervention

Education is also very important. If the individual with ADHD understands what ADHD is and realizes the benefits of his condition, he can better find success. Those that do not understand what is happening have little chance of having improved self esteem and may even fight behavior and medication treatments that are looking to improve his condition.

Understanding And Treating ADHD

A combination of all of these treatment methods is usually the best course of action for the person that has ADHD. Although many parents fight the thought of medications, it is often a necessary part of allowing the child to find success with his condition. No matter who the individual is, help can be found for ADHD in the way of treatments when all aspects of the situation are taken into consideration.

ADHD Treatments: Medication Treatments

ADHD treatments often include some form of treatment medication. There are several medications on the market that are used extensively to help children as well as adults who have been diagnosed with treatment. Many of these treatment options are subject to the individual's reaction to them. Sometimes this means that you will have to try several before finding the right choice for your condition. Finding the right medication means that ADHD can be less of a problem for the individual and they can improve their day to day functions, especially at school or work.

Most medications for ADHD are stimulants. Many individuals do not understand this as many that suffer from ADHD are quite wound up and worked up. Yet, unlike those that would take a stimulant to give them more energy, the stimulants work in a different way for the person with ADHD. They work by stimulating the brain in a specific area to help them to gain benefits such as better attention spans, more control instead of impulse decisions and more focus in the tasks they need to accomplish. These medications work by helping the brain to have greater self regulation.

Here are some of the most common medications for ADHD treatments.

Methylphenidate: These are found in Ritalin, Metadate, Methylin and Focalin. These are usually taken three times per day after meals. There are others including Ritalin LA and Focalin XR that are long doses that will extend up to 12 hours.

Amphetamines: Here, you may find choices such as Dexedrine that is taken several times per day, ADDerall which is both available in short and longer periods and others.

Other medications for ADHD treatment including Atomoxetine, Bupropion which is more well known as Wellbutrin, Benzphetamine which is much less powerful, Provigil which is a new choice, and Clonidine.

There is a lot of trial and error that goes into the determination of the right medication for an individual that suffers from ADHD. The best tool that can be provided to them is accurate diagnosis as well as diligence at taking the medications. When something is not correct with the

Understanding And Treating ADHD

medication, they should let their doctor know right then and there so that an alternative can be found. ADHD treatments with medication should also be helped with behavior and educational help as well. The combination can allow children and adults to find more answers to their questions and overall better results to their needs.

ADHD Treatments: What Happens When Medications Are Not Enough?

Many times, individuals with ADHD do not respond well enough with the medications to offer them enough control and guidance over their situation. When this is the case, everyone involved can become quite frustrated and worried. Yet, there is little doubt that having the right tools and the right education about the condition can help you to get the success you need in finding the right ADHD treatment.

Sometimes, medication is not the only answer available. While any child ore adult that is taking medication for ADHD should never stop taking it unless they talk to their doctor first, it can be quite beneficial to ADD other types of treatments to the fold as well. It is common for there to be differences in one patient to the next, so your first task in helping someone to get through ADHD problems is to find a successful and experienced doctor. All to often the family doctor is the one left to make the decisions about ADHD with the child. Finding someone that specializes can make the medication and the behavior choices better for them.

In Addition, when medications do not seem to be enough treatment for ADHD, it is also important to consider stress levels, emotional trauma (some children with ADHD are depressed or otherwise facing anxiety that can worsen the symptoms) as well as diet. All of these things can trigger increased ADHD symptoms that can make the medications seem as if they are not working enough. Yet, these situations can be treated as well.

Alternate Treatments

There are several alternative treatments to ADHD medications. Those that do not want their child to take medication or do not feel that they want to take them themselves can use these alternative options to offer some help. Some studies have found that those that do not eat a balanced diet that is rich in minerals and vitamins are more likely to experience ADHD. In Addition, there are those treatments which are not proven but can be helpful. Some claim that drinking mild stimulant products like Caffeine filled drinks can provide some of the calming effects of ADHD medications. There are herbal supplements that are available that also encourage help for ADHD.

Understanding And Treating ADHD

It is true that sometimes medication do not work well enough for the individual. That does not mean, though that there is not any treatment or help for them. Working with a doctor that is skilled in the field can offer more success in finding the right solution for the child. There are many theories and misunderstandings out there. Yet, with the skilled doctor, you can find the treatment options that are right for you.

ADHD Treatments: The Diet

When considering the right ADHD treatment for a child or an adult, it can be important to take a look at their specific diet. Those that find that medication do not work, do not want to take medication or are looking for Added benefits with the medications should take a look at the diet of the individual that has ADHD. Studies have shown that many individuals that have ADHD also have diet deficiency. Other studies have shown that some individual's that do have ADHD have a body chemistry that reacts to some food products in the wrong way, leading to worsened symptoms.

It is essential to take a good look at the diet of the individual and adjust it if at all possible. Diet modification can help to improve the ADHD that an individual has, improving their life quality and lessening symptoms. One of the most well known types of diets to consider is that of the Feingold Diet. In this diet, the idea is to pull out some of the most unnatural of elements that are commonly found in food today. This may including such things as salicylates, food colorings and flavors that are not naturally there, as well as preservatives that are not natural.

Modifying the diet can be quite troublesome to individuals that face ADHD. Many times, children are the hardest hit by this change. Removing foods that are packed with preservatives, artificial flavorings and other poor quality ingredients can be difficult as it is in many of the children's favorite foods. The more that they consume of these products though, the more troublesome their health and their ADHD can be.

One effective method to getting past this problem is to keep the diet in mind as a food change for the entire family. As none of these ingredients has shown to be good for the body, everyone can benefit by not consuming things like junk food chips, cookies, and other candies. Limiting them can also be helpful. Working to incorporate better health benefiting products is also a good thing.

There are some studies that show that improving the diet of a child with more whole foods, including foods that are not processed or refined can help to improve their ADHD symptoms. Although it is not thought of as causing the ADHD in the first place, there is evidence that an improved diet can lead to improvements overall for the child or adult that suffers from ADHD.

The Bad Side Of ADHD Treatments

Once a child is diagnosed with ADHD, treatment options will present themselves. Since there are more and more children being diagnosed each day with this condition, there is little doubt that there are going to be some times when the wrong treatment is presented to the child. It is essential that parents take a great deal of caution in dealing with these issues. The best way to do that is to insure that you are fully educated when it comes to ADHD as well as the medications that are provided to the individual. With education about the bad side of ADHD treatments, the right treatment can be beneficial without Added problems.

Side Effects

One thing that needs to be considered is the fact that there are side effects to many of the medications that are used to treat ADHD. Most drugs will have some side effects, but some are much worse than others. While your doctor will tell you the specific side effects for your particular medication, there are some that are more common in these medications. For example, some children have a loss of appetite while the medications are in their systems. Other symptoms that can be common include insomnia, nervousness, weight loss, problems with coming off the medications and mood swings. ADHD medication side effects offer a wide range of benefits and often these benefits can outweigh the side effects of the drug.

Getting Help

When you feel that the side effects of a treatment are troublesome talk to your doctor. He or she may recommend that the dosage of the medications be increased or lowered. Some medications affect some children different. There are several different types of medications that can be used to treat ADHD though. So if one medication is not working well or the side effects are troublesome, your doctor should be contacted as there are other solutions.

Parents of children that are newly diagnosed with ADHD should pay close attention to the medications that the child takes. Sometimes it can take several days for the medication to enter the blood stream enough to see a difference. Sometimes not enough medication is prescribed. In Addition, parents should keep track of any drastic changes or anything that is bothersome or worrisome in their child. With this information they can work closely with their child's doctors to find the most effective dose of medication. Include your child's teachers in this process as well.

ADHD Treatments With Rewards

There are many beliefs about ADHD treatments and what will and will not work for the child. No matter if your child begins to take medications for their condition or not, there are likely to be benefits to the child's behavior if they are able to work with a reward program. These are programs that are designed to help a child to realize that some actions will result in negative reactions from you and that when they do good things that good things lead to positive responses from you. Children that have ADHD need constant reminding of these goals as well as the means to put in place a system that is consistent.

To help your child to learn how to control his behavior, there are several things that you can do.

- Set up a program that will reward your child for good behavior. Determine what the reward is and communicate with the child about what they can do to get that reward.
- Determine a system of punishment that is clear and consistent. A series of warnings that lead to the same punishment each time will help them to recognize what bad behavior leads to.
- Punishments can including removing of various privileges that the child enjoys. In Addition, it can include anything but should be consistent each time the child does the negative behavior.
- The things that are negative behavior should be clearly defined. What things will lead to the punishment? This will help to encourage the realization that poor behavior leads to this punishment.
- Rewards should be provided immediately. Things like words of encouragement, positive reinforcement through spending one on one time together or a special prize are all rewards that can be appropriate.
- Different levels of rewards can be included.

Often times there are goals set forth for the child to accomplish. By having a chart or other mechanism in place where the child can visually see their progress will be helpful as well. This is common done in the form of a chart that allows them to place a check mark or other mark when they accomplish their goal. They can work up the chart to achieve the previously set forth goal then.

When rewarding and punishment programs are put in place, consistency is in place as well. With that comes the clear understanding of what the consequences are and this can help the child to cope with their ADHD. This type of behavior program is often encouraged for the child as confusing discipline can lead to more aggravation on everyone's part.

Finding The Right ADHD Treatment And Doctor

Today, there are more and more children diagnosed with ADHD. This trend does not mean, necessarily that there are more children that have this condition, but more diagnosing is happening now, where it was not just a few years ago. The problem with this is that often times the wrong diagnosis is given. Doctors that are prescribing medications are often not specialists in this field and that alone can lead to problems as there are many products on the market and research is constantly changing. If you or your child has been told that they have ADHD what are you to do to insure that they are getting the best overall treatment for their condition? There are several key elements to take into consideration here.

Consider ADHD Clinics

There are some wonderful clinics available around the country that offers specialists that will work with your child to determine what is causing their ADHD if possible and then to provide for the very best treatment for your child or for you. There are many adults that find this to be the most effective means of solving ADHD questions as these specialists will work with the individual until a solution is finally met.

Clinics often specialize in ADHD and that along allows them to have the latest information, the latest medications and the most knowledge about the subject. In Addition, they are better capable of finding the right solution and the right ADHD treatment faster than others. This can be an ideal way to find the help needed for ADHD suffers.

Consider Schools

In Addition to clinics, there are also specialized schools for children that suffer from ADD or ADHD. When a child is put into this type of environment, they may be more likely to learn in the correct manner. This is due to the way in which lessons are taught. Children with ADHD often learn better in more unique learning environments such as more hands on methods. Although they learn the same things, they also learn how to properly cope with their ADHD as part of the learning process, allowing them to learn how to handle social situations.

Finding the proper ADHD treatment as well as the right doctor for your child is essential in the process to helping them find relief for their ADHD. With many resources available today, there is no doubt that there is help out there. It is just a matter of finding the right help for them.

ADHD Treatments: Is Your Child's Diet A Factor?

There is growing concern about what children are eating and how it affects their lives and their health. Today, children with ADHD are being studies to determine if in fact their diets have something to do with their ADHD. The facts seem to offer that those children that are facing ADHD treatments are missing the boat. That is, while doctors are prescribing medications, there may be some help in providing help to these children through diet modifications. Although there is no way to know for sure what is causing your child's ADHD, it is believed that some children face the symptoms of ADHD because of what they eat.

There are several things that are being considered. Research has shown that children that limit or monitor their intake of certain foods while insuring that the right nutrients are provided can find relief from ADHD without the harmful side effects of medications. Some doctors encourage their patients to work with monitoring diet as well as taking medications. In either case, there is more and more evidence that shows that what your child is consuming is not helping his ADHD.

Some of the most common theories that have shown at least some benefit to those children that have ADHD include the following:

- Limiting the amount of sugar in the child's diet will help to reduce ADHD symptoms.
- Limiting the amount of refine carbohydrates can help this includes white breads and pastas.
- A diet that offers higher amounts of protein that is lean can be helpful.
- Removing foods that the child has even slight allergens or sensitivities to can b helpful.
Here, there is a need for testing to insure that all have been removed from his diet.
- Removing all food Additives from the diet.
- Insuring that the child does not have any heavy metal toxicity and removal of any possible toxins.
- Treatment for any type of bacteria or parasites that the child may have in his intestines.

With the combination of these factors, some researchers believe that the signs and the symptoms of ADHD will be gone. Although you should never stop giving your child is medications without first talking to your doctor, improving the quality of the foods that he eats can be effective at offering some treatment for his condition.

10 Advantages Of Having ADD

Even as the human brain afflicted by ADD does get affected adversely at times, it can still function well enough for persons to benefit from the condition, such as:

1. ADD endows persons affected by this disorder to have an increased sense of empathy since the condition grants them enhanced ability to focus on others and varied view points.

2. A sense of ingenuity is granted by the condition also and many creative people such as artists, movie makers, composers and performing artists besides sculptors have been endowed with increased capabilities, thanks to ADD; Beethoven and Mozart are prime examples of ADD afflicted people being successful.

3. Increased eagerness and motivation towards likeable tasks grips ADD-afflicted persons to perform well on the job if they have the right tools and make a success of it, too.

4. Research has shown that persons assumed to have ADD are blessed with a greater ability to solve puzzles, problems and theories defying explanations so as to keep at it till a logical, correct conclusion is reached; it was the case with famous inventors like .Thomas Edison and Thomas Jefferson.

5. Another advantage of having ADD is getting the Added ability to focus more on reaching goals and meeting short or long term objectives such as living out dreams and keeping jobs, if kept under strict control.

6. Another positive feature of having ADD is that not only does a controlled condition ensure work gets done well, but also endow ADDers with a jovial nature, giving them the ability to laugh and make people around them join in the merriment with their improved sense of humor; in fact, some famous comedians attributed with ADD include Whoopi Goldberg and Robin Williams.

7. A resilient spirit is also attributed to people diagnosed with ADD.

8. Increased intuitiveness thanks to a higher sense of awareness is the Additional gift of ADD, find people diagnosed with this disorder. This ability to think and act faster than others gives

people having ADD the ability to get a deeper insight into the human mind and become more intensely responsive to situations and people around them. Thus, having ADD turns out to be a valuable gift for many such persons with ADD.

9. Innovative thinking and ideation are other abilities that ADD-ers are endowed with, which helps ADD to the strength of a brain-storming session.

10. A Unique perspective thanks to a special ability to look at the world around them is the last but not least important attribute of people afflicted with ADD; while others may not fully understand this advantage, many ADD-ers feel this enables them to share a certain special wavelength with other kindred souls.

Difference Between ADD And ADHD

Many people get confused over ADD and ADHD but learning about the differences between the two conditions helps to lift the common misconceptions about the 2 distinctly different disorders and the nature of each one of them. ADD is a complex condition known as Attention Deficit Disorder, which may have a physiological beginning but multifarious results may arise due to it while ADHD is the short-form of Attention Deficit Hyperactive Disorder with consequences such as increased activity and greater impulse-prone decisions taken by the person suffering it.

Noticeable hyperactivity is apparent to the observant person studying the affected person diagnosed with ADHD. On the other hand, persons suffering from ADD typically have reduced powers of concentration, but there are still various sub-types to both conditions that characterize the problems of the disorders. Some of these are given below:

For example, many readers will recall the common picture of an ADD afflicted person being associated with the image of a small boy bouncing off walls and driving educationists and care-givers batty. The stereotyping for ADHD is easier to identify since it is less difficult to define as compared to the more complicated condition of ADD: it is responsible for causing disturbances in the classroom and other associations set-backs in a group environment and is easier to pick up also. The sad part about ADD though, is that it has many negative side-effects even in the instance of the condition being less visible.

If not attended to urgently, an ADD afflicted person may seem unnaturally 'spaced-out' or disoriented to onlookers, which is really not the case but only look to be so as in the case of an ADD-er gazing out the window with nothing apparent to others to look at! This makes ADD a difficult condition to diagnose and thus many potential patients may go many years without proper treatment as diagnosis has not been reached, giving them the reputation of 'not being all there.'

The result of this lack of timely diagnosis and subsequent missing out on treatment for ADD may cause the mind to drift, which is no less disconcerting for a person suffering the condition. Besides this, the common belief about ADHD was that it only affected boys, which is a myth that has recently been busted: experts reveal even girls can be affected by attention deficit disorder and it may carry on till they reach middle age! However, one major difference is that girls

Understanding And Treating ADHD

afflicted with ADD seem to record the inattentive type of this condition, which is why it has been misdiagnosed frequently as depression. It may also have something to do with the fact that inattentive ADD causes less noticeable problems for the person suffering it and since there is minimal disruption to people around them, many ADD-ers may suffer in silence, without treatment, for years at end, thus Adding to their misery.

This is also the reason why it is imperative for proper treatment to take place that both these limiting disorders are accurately diagnosed in the initial stages and academic situations are the best bet for zoning in on implications of either disorder; then, be it ADD or AHDH, interrupted or incomplete school work will not be an issue and subsequently, timely diagnosis will help parents keep a watchful eye over wards with academic, psychological and general problems. From issues of peer socialization to lack of orderliness to inability to sit still for even short periods or mood swings (quiet to talkative), there are many indications of ADD or ADHD that observant parents can watch out for and get help with if their children show these telling signs indicating either disorders so as to get best scope of treatment from timely counseling and therapy.

Thus, it can be concluded that for a child's complete wellness program to succeed, one must concentrate equally on the psychological as well as the physical aspects of the child's upkeep.

Is Attention Deficit Disorder Actually A Learning Disability?

Attention Deficit Disorder deals with a dysfunctional aspect of a person who may combine other disabilities as well and thus a child affected by this condition will have a good learning process that works for him much like other human beings who can memorize and retain information; their only problem is having a short attention span so attracting and holding their interest for a sustained period of time is crucial for helping their minds retain facts.

Such a child may typically have a problematic academic record but with timely diagnosis and proper treatment, grades in school and concentration power can shoot up, improving performance and productivity for the ADD-er who may have had a bumpy start to educational life; results, however, may differ from individual to individual.

In very young kids (pre-schoolers mostly), there may be other disabilities exhibited that usually include one or more of the following: auditory problems(limited understanding of sounds and words), speech problems, difficulty with the '3 R's (reading, 'riting and 'rithmetic) besides spelling problems. As is the case of Dyslexia (a reading disorder), ADD is very common in kids too who have limitations in learning though it is not necessarily true for all ADD-ers to have the above problems.

Parents and care-givers, including teachers, can help ADD-er kids to improve their learning habits and performance in school by guiding them along lines of having a timetable and daily schedule so as to better utilize their time efficiently and thus improve memory and diligence to activities through careful planning and focus on routine things. This is based on the idea of repetition, which includes keeping things in order, in pre-determined places so its easy to locate them and organize papers in binders, folders and files so they are sorted out easily, reducing time and labor besides being daily planning aids.

The cheerful classroom attitude of a teacher with an inter-active manner can also help children with ADD improve performance as opposed to mere lecturing that can be taken as criticism, since this approach encourages a child to pay attention and reduce distractions so success becomes a habit due to high degree of motivation and understanding offered to the ADD-er.

ADD And Kids

In order to understand ADD in girls better, we can take the example of those tagged as Tomboys as this category of girls most frequently displays the common symptoms associated with ADD such as preferring more physical activities that may be less adventurous as those pursued by boys but no less challenging in terms of exertion required; the consequences are typically that observers find them less inclined towards studies due to their apparent disinterest in and staying organized. Thus, this strong chance of ADD in girls goes undiagnosed for the simple reason that it is overlooked.

The other category of girls that go unnoticed as being potential ADD sufferers belong to the talkative segment, who exhibit a certain tendency to chattiness, which combines increased period of activity and certain dull periods, so on the whole, these girls seem extroverts. At times, even strict warnings do not prevent ADD affected girls from continuing to talk and besides being inclined towards telling stories in details, they can also stray from one topic to another due to this condition.

The third kind of girls suffering from ADD are those categorized as Daydreamers, who talk less and seldom draw attention to themselves, but cannot seem to pay adequate in class; they are in sharp contrast with their 'chatty' counterparts, who are also suffering from ADD, but a different form which is manifested differently too! This last kind of ADD afflicted girls may exhibit signs of worry and sadness when assigned school work as they have limited attention and their thoughts tend to stray. Many may also suffer from a lack of understanding on the part of parents and school teachers who are likely to attribute this lack of staying power in the ADD-girls to being indolent or disorderliness. Thus, it is very important to diagnose ADD in time and accurately for children to get proper and timely help and treatment.

Girls affected by ADD are a considerable number and some may even have an impressive IQ rate so as to qualify them as being 'Gifted;' yet even as they may not lag behind in school work, these children can suffer other ADD related problems that prevent them from having a fulfilling life as an adult. This is why it is crucial to educate parents about the true nature of ADD and that it is different from a learning disorder as children may be great performers in school but unable to face challenges of a regular lifestyle that is important for healthy, mature and organized living

Understanding And Treating ADHD

in the real world. ADD affected children have lesser ability to deal with school work after high school academic levels and the symptoms of ADD become more apparent after this stage.

If ADD goes undiagnosed, it can mean needless agony for a child being tagged disorganized, stupid or plain lazy for no fault of theirs and they may suffer silently for years or worse still, suffer from low self esteem, become quitters, or depressed; thus, identification and treatment for ADD is very important at the early stages to prevent and control the disorder.

Adult ADD: 5 Tips For Job Effectiveness

1. Pick a Career with Passion! A profession that one is enthusiastic about is one that is more likely to sustain their interest and motivation levels, resulting in greater sense of accomplishment that is necessary to maintain their sense of involvement as compared to a job they are less keen or knowledgeable about. A Job chosen with some passion has more of a chance in establishing success through pleasurable working attitudes and thus, ADD-ers are advised to look for their best jobs this way.

2. Stick to a Structured Environment! Those ADD-ers working for themselves need to know the significance of working in a structured, organized environment as much as their work outside home counterparts, who are employed at companies and have work plans and timetables sorted out for themselves by managers etc. Self employed ADD affected persons have as much a responsibility towards deciding work timings, off days and sticking to these in a disciplined manner as company employed ADD-ers as this particular factor is decisive in meriting them completed projects on timely basis besides meeting targets objectively and successfully each time.

3. The Devil lies in the Details: an important aspect for work success that all ADD-ers need to pay attention to! This is a very important point for all ADD-ers to remember as paying attention to particulars and specifics is a crucial aspect of generating success with problem solving, innovation, ideation, lead generation etc, all of which are contributes towards making them good organizers and efficient workers, especially at executive-level jobs. For the self-employed ADD-ers, there may be a better chance of succeeding at their chosen profession if they hire Additional support at the work-place even if the proposition seems a tad expensive as in the long run, an associate can provide valuable help in terms of business rules and targets being met besides sharing work load at crucial times. Company employees suffering ADD should pass on details of the work in hand to other executive co-workers or responsible associates who can ADD value to the assignment and prevent build-up of back-log.

4. Time management is of utmost importance to an ADD-er: not just day-to-day planning, but when to plan is also crucial! Time to plan may take 15 minutes as in the case of making a to-do list; this can be done before leaving for work or when winding up the work day, whichever is a more convenient time personally for the ADD-er; however, it is important that planning be done and regular updation of the to-do list be incorporated too. This includes updating calendars and fragmenting important work assignments that make be tackled in stages to make it less formidable and easier to deal with effectively, thereby increasing productivity.

5. Stop being finicky! Excessively being obsessed with doing a perfect job will just bring on heartache for yourself and can actually put off a lot of people from tackling a project report or paper each time they look at the task to be tackled, resulting in disinterest and consequent lack of the job getting done at all. Thus, knowing the difference between a job well done and a perfect job is very essential for ADD-ers who need to focus on putting in best efforts in a timely, organized and structured way instead of concentrating on perfection, which is elusive in this world anyway.

An Introduction To Attention Deficit Disorder

Among one of the most misdiagnosed brain disorders, ADD or Attention Deficit Disorder, is a condition that is an unpalatable reality for many people; the lack of proper information about this neurological limitation results in many sufferers having to suffer even more indignity and lack of understanding from family and friends, which is why it is important to learn and understand much about ADD so as to be able to identify a person affected by it and treat them respectfully. This article is meant to be an introduction to ADD and records valuable facts about it, including nature, diagnosis methods, assorted means of treating ADD and is aimed at being a tool for understanding the scope of ADD affected lives.

ADD or ADHD (Attention Deficit Hyperactivity Disorder) as it is sometimes referred to, is the condition of limited attention span suffered for a prolonged time by the person affected by this neurological disorder; it manifests itself in various forms such as motor restlessness and impulsiveness displayed by patients with nearly 4.4% of adults possessing a certain degree of ADD, suggests medical research.

ADD, as we understand it, is a problem related to the brain dysfunction or limitation as such, that is a result of malfunctioning of its dopamine neurotransmitter systems; it is typically linked with hereditary factors, which makes it a strong probability for a child with a parent or close relative with ADD to also share the disorder and its adversities. As far as twins are concerned, ADD has a stronger chance (50%) of occurring in the second child if one has been diagnosed with it. While the earlier viewpoint about causes of ADD were mainly linked to poor nutritional habits, recent scientific research dismisses this claim as being incorrect and prefers to deal in a like manner with other myths about ADD occurring, such as allergy, inadequate parenting measures or drugs etc. The medical experts of today lay more emphasis on ADD having been caused due to intense head injury, a fetallead alcohol syndrome, lead toxicity cases and even thyroid irregularities which they feel need to be completely ruled out as probable causes before a person is attributed with having ADD.

Being diagnosed with ADD means that the person is receiving an insufficient supply of neuro-chemicals, which simply means proper stimulation to the brain cells is missing and this results in the brain having to find other ways to release these chemicals. This is why individuals with ADD are prone to being involved in excessive physical activity, movements and situations that require them to stimulate their brains in an enhanced manner so as to meet this challenge, but it is not always a conscious decision on their part rather, it is a relfex action for them.

Among the chief disadvantages caused to people suffering from ADD due to the hyperactivity levels is that they are ill-equipped mentally and physiologically to deal with demanding circumstances that may not necessarily appeal to them or their level of activity; thus, issues like school work that are less than stimulating may actually be off-putting for ADD-ers and is likely to get adversely affected with the child suffering low grades and rebukes from teachers. A story based on the times when information about ADD was scarce goes along these lines: an ADD affected kid would suddenly get up on his desk when the class was being conducted and start telling jokes, humoring everyone much to the chagrin of those present and though his attempt was purely to be entertaining and people initially though it humorous, he did come to be regarded as a disturbing element. However, soon it was realized that the child suffered from ADD and these actions were actually beyond his control. Others who are not so lucky to be understood as being identified with ADD can suffer serious consequences of this disorder, including damage to personal relationships, lack the ability to be permanently employed and suffer depression or get involved with dubious activities just to stimulate themselves, which can also have legal consequences.

Attention Deficit Disorder: Is It A Disease Or Just A Phase?

Think back to your childhood: were you full of beans and running about for no reason at all sometimes? Did you often lose interest in what you were doing and get distracted easily or have trouble sitting still in one place? Short attention span, inability to concentrate for long on one thing or activity and focusing on simply doing certain things are all elements of being youthful, which many people will remember; however, this lack of reflecting on doing things and simply going ahead with impulses is now being re-defined by science as something beyond the scope of a simple childhood. We see what it now being looked upon as:

Not really thinking about the reasons or consequences of an action and exhibiting the above traits is now being regarded as less than normal by the medical fraternity, which has coined a phrase called ADD or Attention Deficit Disorder, which is a result of a neurological imbalance, but not really a disease as such.

Many doctors and psychologists are still not in agreement over a person having ADD merely based on certain commonalities; some experts associated with the mental health association demanded a proper method and scientific tools to help categorize individuals diagnosed with ADD and ways to identify this condition with fool-proof measures. This meant ascertaining a certain brain deficiency and though ADD was studied as an apparent dysfunction in a group of people suffering from encephalitis, (an inflammation of the brain), it is no longer a measure for determining ADD. Thus, even persons with no brain deficiencies are also classified under the heading of ADD affected individuals today.

There are 2 kinds of ADD: one with hyperactivity and the other, without; the former is also referred to as ADHD where due to the hyperactivity, the person may refuse to stay motionless for a period of time, exhibit impulsive behavior such as excessive talking, physical activity, impatience with situations or even be unable to play peacefully. They also have a tough time concentrating on simple tasks at hand and get easily distracted.

Thus, even with nearly 3-5 % persons diagnosed with ADD, there is a need to know more about this condition, which is neither a phase nor a disease but a medical condition that requires counseling for early diagnosis, accurate and timely treatment and to help make the ADD-er a successful, balanced and capable person. At times, outward signs of ADD may not be present

Understanding And Treating ADHD

and therefore the condition can be difficult to diagnose but with proper check-ups and tools, the mannerisms and undesirable behavior of ADD can be toned down and controlled considerably.

Therefore, a combination of various symptoms, ADD which can generate many problems, both psychological and mental besides careless behavior, should be treated in a timely manner by experts in the medical field so as to grant genuine and timely help to the sufferers for whom living with ADD is a harsh reality, not just a phase in life. It is a mistaken belief to assume that people with ADD are not suffering and its just a bundle of indications; ADD-ers require understanding, support and treatment and its wrong to expect them to simply snap out of it as its not a stage, but a reality.

Attention Deficit Disorder: Is It Really That?

ADD is the abbreviated form of a neurological disorder that mostly affects boys during the elementary schooling stage; it has certain marked symptoms such as reduced concentration span, restlessness, careless actions and inattention to details exhibited by those affected. However, in order to determine the cause of these symptoms and the validity of the condition so as to bring about correct treatment, it is important to learn about the true nature of ADD and what it means for the individual and that's what this article deals with.

Sometimes, specific signs of ADD may be present on the surface and at others, a more intense form of this psychological problem may manifest itself in the form of depression, arrested brain development, bipolar disorders or extreme nervousness, but the infrequent or occasional occurrence of a spell of inattentively should never hastily be judged as ADD as it can be an allergic reaction, nutritional deficiencies or even due to environmental sensitivity or even excess caffeine in the diet.

The many possibilities besides ADD are also the reason why many a time physically active and energetic boys are misdiagnosed with having ADD when they exhibit generally adventurous behavior, short attention spans in school, changing thoughts and high bursts of energy, which are generally associated with ADD. Since most school-going kids are keenly tuned in to TV programs in the upward range of 40+ hours a week or computer games, its natural that a lot of energy is saved up so can be easily directed towards activities, not necessarily indicating ADD.

In order to determine whether the suspected condition is actually ADD, mannerisms such as high creativity, ideation, being gifted or being visually innovative should be analyzed.

This high aptitude in a child suspected of having ADD must be properly studied, especially for those kids with short attention spans and those displaying agitation frequently; they may be treated with Dexerdine or Ritalin medicine but since these can have dangerous side-effects, they are only a temporary measure not a cure.

A child's parents need to be alert and focused on the behavior of their kid in order to accurately look for and find the absolute mannerisms indicative of ADD existing in the child so as to get him or her the best treatment through timely, accurate diagnosis.

Attention Deficit Disorder: Getting Your Facts Right

A lot has been written about ADHD, which is a common disorder today but the many stereotypes of the naughty brat running out in a crazy fashion or spoiling everything in his way are more misconceptions than the rule for those suffering this neurological limitation and its not always that simple to spot a child with ADD even when we think we can do so on an outing. The common misconception of the unruly, bad boy belies the fact that even the withdrawn and silent little girl may be affected equally by ADD, which manifests itself in various forms and thus needs a proper introduction for those unaware of the scope of this condition.

In reality, ADD can be manifested in many forms: from the quiet to the overly chatty, from those almost afraid to speak up to those completely disinterested in responding to conversations and even the most physically active to a silent, brooding type, thus, diagnosing ADD may be difficult at times. However, some obvious signs of diagnosing ADD are present for the keen observer: these include checking for a person with limited ability to focus, stay attentive for a period of time, inability to remember things and individual suffering low self esteem, those tuning out of a conversation to those persons being extremely disorganized.

Some of the disadvantages a person with ADD can suffer include not being able to follow conversations, being incapable of functioning in a structured manner and limited attention span which typically results in their having arrested mental development so school work is adversely affected as project deadlines are seldom met due to lack of time management or ability to manage personal belongings and tasks with an organized outlook and time-keeping.

Symptoms of ADD also include an inordinate lack of energy, increased laziness, giving more importance to others, being under-assertive and downright door-mats to being too polite and avoiding crowded places as a result of being excessively shy, therefore socially withdrawn even as ADD-ers do manage to build bonds a few times, though not always.

ADD in girls is largely overlooked as this species is assumed be naturally shy and therefore ADD-er girls can be left untreated for a long time, which is a bad thing. From quietness that is not actually demureness to excessive humility that is misinterpreted over politeness, ADD affected girls are very sensitive and react emotionally to criticism, struggling to cope with life in a silent way and oft times, being stressed by this too. However, their ADHD counterparts are considerably less affected by tiredness or stress factors such as caused by criticism and therefore sail through life effortlessly while the ADD affected girls suffer in silence and sometimes retreat into a shell as a result.

To help a person with ADD, it is important to understand that girls affected by this disorder are not only emotional, but also prone to being overly impulsive, sensitive and hyper-active whether they are extroverts or introverts. This raises their normal stress levels, which need to be managed through various techniques that can be taught to them at early on in life to prevent and control the condition from causing them long-term developmental damage or limiting their life as an adult. It is referred to as the revival time to regroup as ADD-ers attempt to collect themselves after an emotionally turbulent time by way of these methods. Even ever-loving parents can be the cause of sending ADD affected girls to the deep end with critical examination of their actions and remarks focusing on their mistakes, such as lack of intelligent action, getting low grades, displaying less than ideal behavior or making wrong decisions that do not appeal to the grown-ups, which can all deflate the affected individual. This kind of criticism must be avoided by well-meaning parents as it can be damaging to the ADD affected girl and a preferable way to dealing with their wards is to offer constructive criticism with advise on practical ways to improve instead of negative commentary that can be damaging to the child's dignity.

Focusing on a girl's particular asset or skill in a particular field or task is preferable to simply criticizing an ADD affected child as whatever limited enthusiasm and motivation the girl may have is lost as a consequence of feelings of worthlessness that creep in with the criticism of elders. Appreciating finer points, boosting their morale and giving positive feedback on their good performance in school is a better and more affective way to get ADD affected girls to develop into confident and worthy individuals.

Attention Deficit Disorder: The Signs And Symptoms

The first thing that may be noticeable about an ADD affected child is the increased level of physical activity, though hyperactivity does not always point to ADD and usually combines other factors such as impulsive behavior, lack of attention or a certain tendency to be distracted.

While being distracted and having a reduced attention span are typical signs of ADD that go hand in hand, other symptoms include having a limited ability to attend to details and not being able to see tasks through till the end, which can even persist for more than six months at a stretch in extreme cases, adversely affecting the daily school work of the child.

Children diagnosed with ADD exhibit impulsive behavior that can manifest itself in many ways, including running away from their desks, getting distracted towards other classroom happenings and losing focus on the task at hand besides given answers to questions that were not asked; all these are common traits of ADD affected kids.

ADD-er kids are also very sensitive to criticism and comments made to them need to be toned down to prevent them getting hurt and too upset to perform productively as this hypersensitivity is a hindrance in letting them concentrate, resulting in poor grades even as they do not exactly have a learning difficultly. Thus, ADD affected kids in particular, need more understanding than regular kids as this low attention span makes them incapable of completing assigned tasks, lowering their schoolwork output.

ADD affected boys are different from girls diagnosed with the same condition: while boys are usually more active, girls exhibit short attention span in class but the similarity is that both sexes are difficult to manage due to unruly behavior they exhibit, which can make them aggressive to the extent of being abusive. However, since all ADD affected children are separate individuals, they should be treated differently for the methods of controlling undesirable behavior and caregivers are advised to consult and verify their aggression and hyperactivity levels as being indicative of ADD by visiting a medical professional as only an expert can diagnose this condition accurately.

Understanding The True Nature Of Attention Deficit Hyperactivity Disorder

ADHD is the abbreviated form of a medical condition known as Attention Deficit Hyperactivity Disorder, which is now recognized as a mental disorder affecting nearly 3-7% of children that can manifest itself through a combination of indications, including disruptive, disobedient and undesirable behavior that is constant and diminishes their quality of life. For this reason, even as the children don't have adequate control over their mental faculties and thus their behavior, it is important to identify and treat ADHD symptoms and the condition, improving their reduced powers of concentration and short attention span.

Besides children, even adults are affected adversely by this mental disorder, called Adult Attention Deficit Disorder or AADD, which can be a result of their having been diagnosed with ADHD as children as almost 30 to 70% of ADHD kids grown up with the reality of having to live with the condition and take counseling help for dealing with it in their daily lives. With timely diagnosis and proper treatment, handling the condition requires less help as the children and young people grow up; the real challenge, then, lies in detecting it early to enable timely, accurate treatment, sometimes through medication also.

ADHD in children has several indications such as lack of concentration power, impulsive behavior and inability to sit still for a period of time, which makes it difficult to diagnose in adults with the same condition, who can exhibit a certain restlessness. This is the reason why adults with AADD have problems in organizing their lives into a structured environment and enjoy sustained success in career and personal life, but it can be achieved through time management and proper counseling for the disorder.

Thus, it is important to understand the true nature of ADHD as being a mental disorder that calls for early, timely and accurate medical help and possible medication that can cure it to the best degree possible to enable the individual diagnosed with it to lead a fulfilling life.

8 Essential Skills For Managing Attention Deficit Disorder

Many adults who have ADD feel overwhelmed at times with regular life chores and responsibilities as they are unable to manage time and errands effectively. This article deals with workable, practical and useful ways that can be incorporated into daily life scheduling in order to bring about an organized, structured and more productive lifestyle for ADD-ers.

Being diagnosed with ADD can be overwhelming for many people who can find it difficult to even attend to routine chores as even these look like obstacles to them; thus, understanding the basics of proper time management is important for them to stay atop things. This includes daily planning done effectively on a regular basis to control stress levels and actually get work done right on time, every time, minimizing hassles all round for ADD-ers.

Sometimes, the day may pass by in a haze for ADD-ers who may have sleepless nights considering they didn't get anything worthy accomplished and simply focusing on their long to-do list that calls for more enthusiasm than they can muster; this may leave them tired, disorganized, lacking creativity, contentment and energy.

These Eight Essential Tips are designed at helping ADD-ers realize and focus on various abilities they can concentrate on in order to improve their lifestyles: take a look!

1. Easing the Pace: is very important for people with ADD as being hyper-active and having a hurried pace only works to wear down limited stores of energy and enthusiasm to start and stick to tasks; thus, slowing down to a comfortable and realistic pace is very important to effectively handle jobs.

2. Setting Aside some 'Me-time': is another important ability ADD-ers need to practice in order to give themselves the importance they are due because their innate tendency to focus on other people's needs may at times deprive them of essential personal time and energy.

3. Learning more about Your own ADD condition: is of utmost important in knowing how to handle it right as this disorder can manifest itself differently for different individuals.

4. Learn to categorize individual methods of learning and processing information that work best results for you as an ADD-er and recognize ones that hinder your concentration abilities or feelings to interfere with enhancing right personal and professional decisions and actions in order to simplify your life.

5. Focus on your strong points and emphasize your key areas of expertise to always stay on top of the world as holding positive thoughts helps realize these into actions with fervent spirit and right efforts, Adding to a sense of accomplishment and raising self-esteem.

6. Be an optimist: as thinking along negative lines only brings down energy, enthusiasm and positive thoughts that can make a success of a task besides holding you down. Charge ahead with positive thinking!

7. Make Time for Time Planning: as daily planning at a fixed time for all tasks, big or small, is essential to the well-being of all ADD-ers who may have difficulty attending to multiple chores, so may need to develop tools and strategies for proper time management and administration in order to ensure good beginnings result in happy and successful endings, including meeting goals.

8. Develop the ability to meet challenges head-on: attempt at stepping out of a comfort zone in order to bring novelty, creativity and higher degrees of motivation towards enhancing the quality of life, whether it means asking for a raise, taking up a new hobby, learning a new skill or finally pursuing a dream.

Planning The Daily Life For Adults With ADD

Those adults who have been diagnosed with ADD or Attention Deficit Disorder as this neurological imbalance is known as in medical circles, will appreciate that attention to details is something they have often felt the lack of; this is not a conscious decision on their part but rather a result of the disorder, even for those who have objectives chalked out mentally and are eagerly waiting to achieve them. However, the sense of wishing themselves out of the efforts required to do the job right is common to all adults with ADD and sometimes this attitude can be overwhelming when they need to focus on starting on any project. Therefore, a few practical tips on time management and workable approaches for enthusiastic beginnings and sticking to the job are more important than simply visualizing the end goal being met, which is what we tackle here.

That adults with ADD find it difficult to begin right is very true in daily living as well as handling careers; this is why it is crucial for them to prioritize right beginnings to ensure happy endings and fruitful ones at that, especially to minimize stress and guilt factors that can lower productivity even with the best intentions when they started out. Here is where a daily planner would help adults with ADD make planning a habit that supports structured and organized thought and action.

Quick tips for developing a daily routine for adults with ADD include setting aside a time to plan, going over the list of tasks and the calendar. While the first helps to get a routine in order be it first thing in the morning or before hitting the sack at night when ADD-ers are at their attentive best, the second helps to review the to-do list, which is essential for organized output and meeting objectives besides acting as a regular reminder for chores that need to be attended to. Then, routinely rewriting ely re-write this list to tick off those already attended to (gives a sense of achievement which helps build up enthusiasm for tackling new tasks) and note down new ones. The most important tasks should ideally head the list and bigger ones can be broken down to multiple steps to make them easy to tackle. Reviewing a calendar is the final step towards organized planning that helps adults with ADD keep up to date with a checklist guiding them for right actions for this day and the next, blocking off appointments on a planner and ensuring commuting time is included in this so the remainder of the day can be planned for other tasks. Just a quarter of an hour kept aside to plan a schedule can thus help adults with ADD tackle everyday situations with ease and lead a hassle-free life.

<u>Understanding The Meaning Of An ADD Diagnosis:</u>
<u>Some</u> <u>Facts!</u>

Nearly 30 years ago, an energetic, lively, highly creative child with enhanced brainpower were upgraded to a higher class if found to be lacking concentration in class-work and showing impulsive, impatient behavior for this was assumed to be a result of the work set to them being less than their level of intelligence; the matter is altogether different today as kids with these traits are termed as ADD affected children. We learn more about diagnosing this condition.

The above mentioned symptoms i.e. impulsive behavior, impatience, disruptive and unruly mannerisms as well as short attention span are associated with the condition known as ADD, or an Attention Deficit Disorder today, which needs immediate treatment for early control.

A new discovery, ADD is most common in primary school boys who are seen as impulsive, restless and highly energetic creatures who have trouble concentrating on school work. They are typically hyperactive kids who can spend 40 + hours watching TV or playing computer games and since this does not really call on huge amounts of energy to be expended by them, they have a lot of it left over for exerting in other activities.

Besides the above symptom, ADD affected kids exhibit distracted behavior due to many reasons, some serious and others not so; at times, this may or may not be a psychological disturbance or reflective of the child's fitness level but a result of child abuse or negligent parenting. Among the methods of treating ADD, there is medical help in the form of Ritalin, a prescription drug, which is also sometimes looked upon as child abuse if used for a long time as it has side-effects.

Among ADD symptoms, there are some forms of manifestation that are of chief concern for physicians, such as ADD that causes psychological problems including bipolar disorder, excessive worrying and depression or brain defects while other instances can be less difficult to deal with and occur in the form of an allergy, environmental sensitivity, nutritional deficiency or due to high dose of caffeine.

Understanding And Treating ADHD

This is why it is very important for an ADD affected child's caregivers to be particular about identifying, diagnosing and treating the condition as early as possible for best results to show through timely and correct medication as well as counseling.

<u>Tips For Parents Looking After A Child With ADD: Useful And Practical</u>

When a child is diagnosed with Attention Deficit Disorder or ADD, it is always an emotionally overwhelming time for the parents who usually realize only then that the child is in need of their understanding, support and proper treatment. From remorse, to feeling a lack of control to empathy for the ADD affected child, the range of emotions for parents can vary and even frustration at the situation is normal to experience: but specialists advise parents never to be disheartened as there are many methods to help them stay atop the situation, impossible as it may seem initially, it is not so.

Here we enumerate some ways that parents can use to help kids cope with ADD:

1. Research the condition in order to have useful and updated information about it - get your ADD facts right! This will help you as parents understand the true nature of the disorder and learn about practical ways to support and care for the ADD affected child as you will better understand the kid's personal situation and problems.

2. Learn about the symptoms, causes, consequences and forms ADD can manifest itself in so as to help your child best besides finding out about the best treatment so you are prepared for dealing with the disorder at every stage in the child's school and personal life; this includes taking medical advice, counseling and medication to improve the situation as and when needed.

3. Always medicate the child affected with ADD only on medical advice, which is essentially a personal choice as many parents are not too keen on using drugs to help children normalize their lives but wish for them to have a structured, organized and productive life through training and behavior modification as well as proper planning to make informed choices and smart decisions.

4. Discussing various kinds of behavioral therapies with the child's counselor is very important to ascertain which one/s apply to your child's specific condition and can help provide your child with the skills to enable better output in terms of energy, efforts and efficiency. Strategies for your child's improved mental health should be carefully guided by your child's current actions

and the consequences you find desirable for him or her; these should be determined by you to instill discipline and define limits for the child.

It has been recognized that a parent is the child's best teacher and motivator, thus, a parent's responsibility is not merely to encourage the child but to ensure an upbringing that supports progress in the school as well as the home. Working closely along side teachers and doctors as a team of caregivers will ensure that every parent whose child is diagnosed with ADD can benefit from well-meaning advice after knowing more details of their ward's conditions and symptoms to devise the best possible developmental program for ADD-ers to have a normal, happy and positive life by emphasizing their self-worth and boosting their morale.

This will ensure children with ADD who often suffer low self-esteem and bouts of depression stay away from negative thoughts and a positive attitude is build up, with timely, mature parental support stemming from love and expert medical help. One vital way of ensuring an ADD affected child gets all the help he or she needs is for the parents to join a support group and reach out to similarly affected families.

Understanding And Treating ADHD

This Product Is Brought To You By

DAVID A OSEI